# Almond Oil - Magic in a Flask

Be As Beautiful On the Outside As You Are Inside

# Disclaimer

No part of this eBook may be reproduced, stored or transmitted in any form or by any means including mechanical or electronic without prior written permission from the author.

While the author has made every effort to ensure that the ideas, guidelines and information presented in this eBook are safe, they should be used at the reader's discretion. The author cannot be held responsible for any personal or commercial damage arising from application or misinterpretation of information presented herein.

# Summary

Are you tired of trying one beauty product after another? Are you frustrated at the empty promises of long hair and beautiful skin? Are you looking for a one stop solution for all your beauty and health problems? If yes then you have come to the right place.

Almond oil is nothing less than a miracle product which will help you in reviving the glow of your skin, the shine of your hair, and beauty of your hands and nails. Almond oil is not only used a beauty product but it can also be used as a substitute for cooking oil, which is one of its many health benefits.

This book will tell you everything that you need to know about the uses and benefits of almond oil. It also includes tips and recipes that will help you incorporate almond oil in your diet.

Read this book till the end and get mesmerized by how almond oil can help you enhance your beauty and maintain a healthier lifestyle.

Enjoy Reading.

## Table of Contents

Be As Beautiful On the Outside As You Are Inside

## Introduction

For hundreds of years, almond oil has been one of the basic ingredients of many beauty products. Experts have pointed out a number of benefits of almond oil, and beauty industry is still unable to grasp all that they can achieve with incorporating almond oil in their beauty products.

With its sweet smell and smooth texture, almond oil offer beauty and health benefits that no other oil does. If you only have almond oil on the list of beauty products that you use, then probably you have all that you need.

Besides being a wondrous beauty product, almond oil has a number of health benefits too. It contains unsaturated fats that not only helps you in controlling the cholesterol levels in your body but also helps in producing good fats that helps your body to produce the energy it requires to stay healthy and fit.

Read along if you are curious about the complete extent of the benefits of almond oil. Learn how to use almond oil to enhance your outer beauty and try out our delicious recipes to improve your inner health.

# Nutritional Facts About Almond Oil

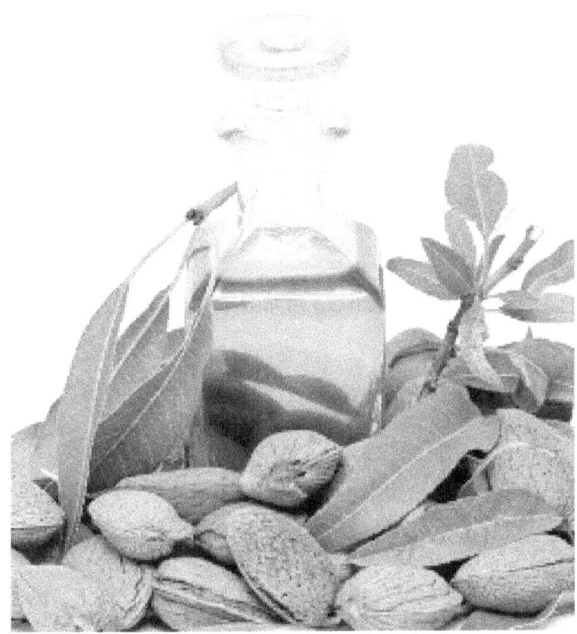

Here are some of the nutritional facts about almond oil to give you an idea of how remarkably beneficial it can be for your beauty and health care.

1. Almond oil contains minerals such as magnesium and calcium.

2. It helps in decreasing cholesterol levels of your body.

3. It also helps in the reduction of LDL (low density lipoproteins) and triglycerides.

4. The quantity of unsaturated fats is high in almond oil.

5. It is cholesterol free.

6. Almond oil contains phytosterols that absorbs the cholesterol of your body.

7. Almond oil is rich in good fats such as polyunsaturated and monounsaturated fats, both of which decrease the probability of heart diseases.

8. It is rich in vitamin E that keeps your skin moisturized and hydrated.

9. Vitamin E also slows down the sign of aging.

10. Almond oil contains Omega-6 helps in strengthening the hair and prevention of hair loss.

11. It makes your hair look silky and shiny.

12. Omega-6 not only makes a person smarter but it also helps in maintaining healthy brain tissues.

13. According to research almond oil is highly effective against diabetes and obesity.

# Almond Oil for Hair

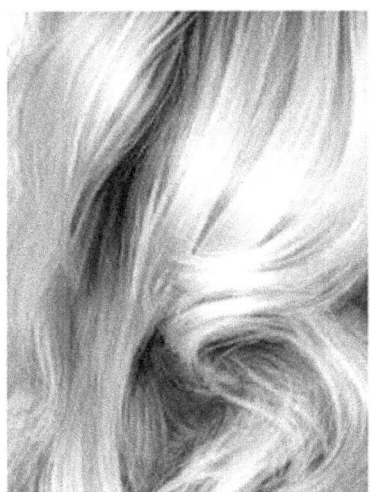

Hair is one of the most distinct features in humans. Having luxurious, beautiful and shiny hair is the dream of every girl.

Having so many hair care products in the market makes it extremely difficult to decide on one product that will answer all your hair concerns. There are only a few products that will deliver on their promise of improving the health of your hair.

However there is one product that is not only suitable for all skin types but also improves the health of your hair drastically and that product is almond oil.

Read along to know how almond oil will help your hair and the different ways in which you can use almond oil.

## Benefits

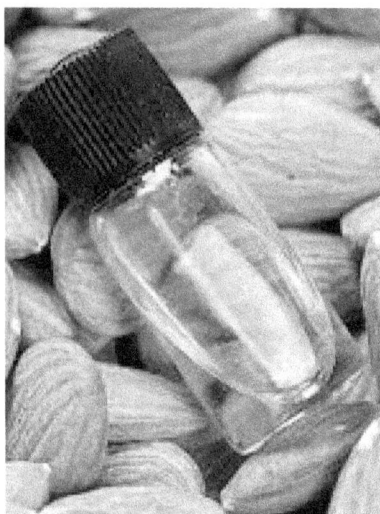

Following is the list of benefits that you can avail by using almond oil or almond oil products for your hair:

1. Almond oil makes your hair soft and manageable by nourishing your hair from cuticles.

2. It repairs the damaged hair and promotes the growth of new and healthy hair.

3. Almond oil strengthens your hair from within, protecting them from damage and breakage.

4. Regular use of almond oil restores the lost luster, and shine of your hair.

5. Almond oil helps in prevention of hair fall.

6. Almond oil also prevents the scalp from getting dry which is one of the main reasons of dandruff.

7. Almond oil will help your scalp hydrated to avoid dandruff issues.

8. Almond oil helps in growth of shiny and healthy hair by keeping your hair follicles conditioned.

9.  Almond oil helps in managing frizzy hair.

10. Almond oil thickens your hair making them stronger and shinier.

11. Almond oil enhances the volume of your hair.

12. Almond oil helps in prevention of split ends.

13. It smoothen your hair making them more attractive.

14. Almond oil curbs skin irritation.

15.  It prevents itching on your scalp.

16. Almond oil has a nice sweet smell that makes your hair smell sweet and fresh.

## Usage Methods

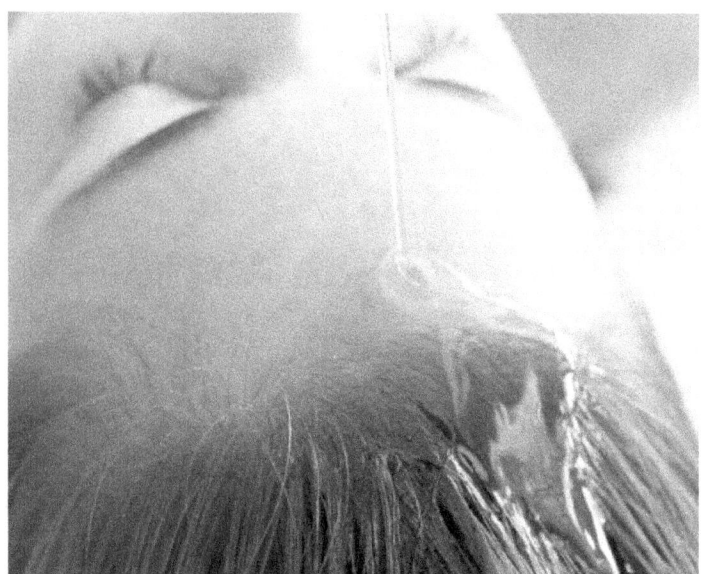

Applying oil to your hair is something that is very traditional and has been done for ages, but there are certain ways of application of oil in your hair that makes it even more effective for the growth and nourishment for your hair. Following are some of the methods that you can employ to apply almond oil in your hair.

## Oil treatment

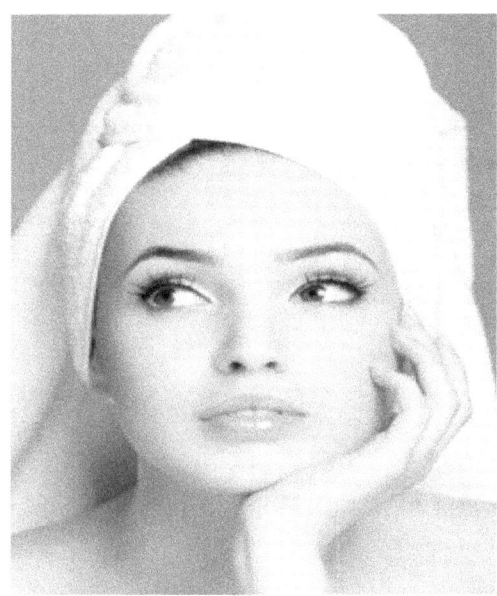

This is the first method of applying almond oil in your hair. In this method you can apply oil directly in your hair and wrap your head with a shower cap or a towel. You can leave oil in your hair for as long as you want. After the oil has stayed in your hair for considerable amount of time (preferably an hour) wash it off with shampoo.

You can apply oil to both dry and damp hair, but make sure that your hair is not dripping wet.

This method is most beneficial if you have a dry scalp because, through this method, oil gets time to sink in your skin. Make sure that you massage your scalp well before you cover your head with towel or shower cap.

## Apply after Shampoo

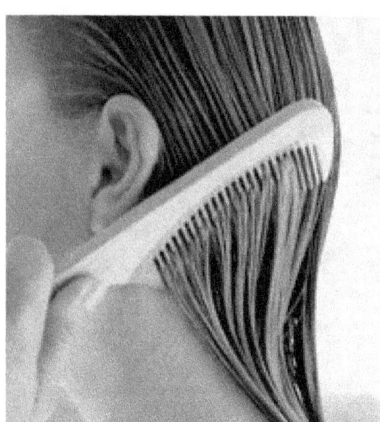

The best way to take advantage of the sealant properties of almond oil is to apply it after you shampoo.

In this method you just take a small amount of almond oil and apply to your hair while they are still damp. After you are done applying, dry your hair and style your hair as you usually do.

Make sure that you take just a small amount of oil as too much oil will weigh down your hair. The best way to ensure that you use little oil is to pour a small amount of oil in your palms, rub your palms together and then run your hands through your scalp.

If you have split ends then applying a small amount of oil to the tips of your hair will be sufficient to control split ends.

## Apply To Styled Hair

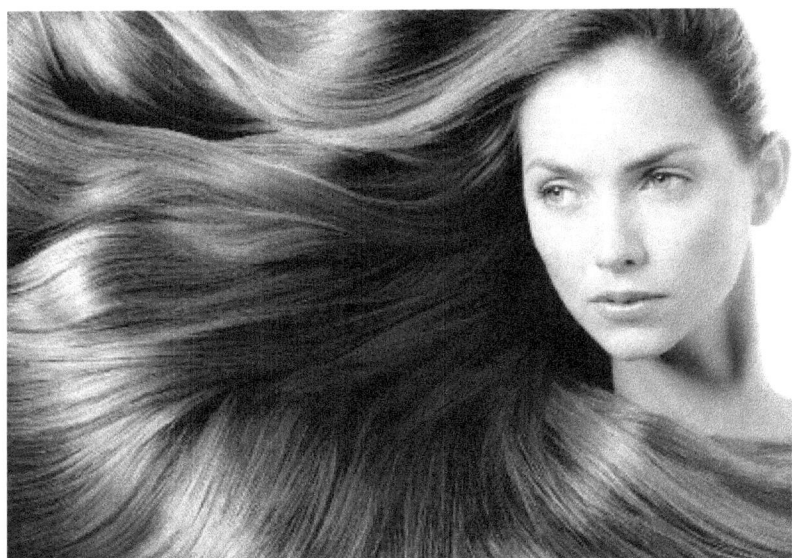

Applying almond oil to your styled hair will make them look shinier. Make sure that you apply a very small amount lightly over your hair. The oil will add luster to your hair.

This method will not only solve your problem of frizzy hair but will also protect your hair from dust and damage.

# Almond Oil for Skin

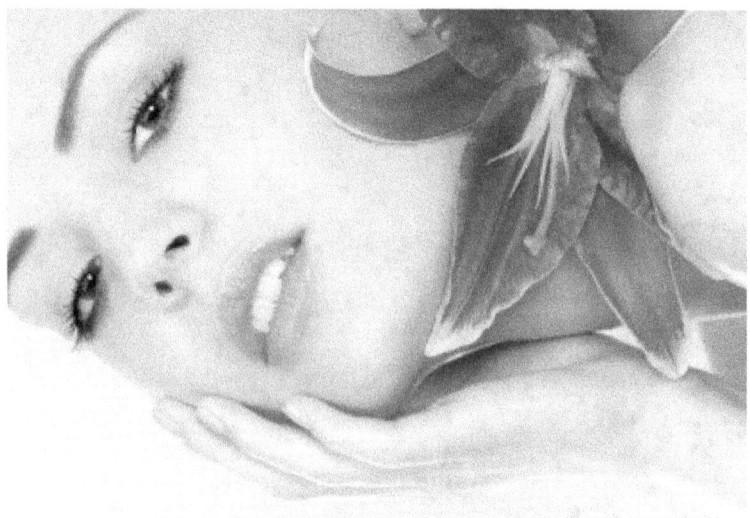

Skin gets the most exposure in human body and therefore it is most difficult to protect. A skin that is not well taken care of shows early signs of aging, uneven skin tones, and is also prone to a number of skin diseases.

There are a number of products in the market that promise to provide ultimate skin solutions and most of them do, but very few products have the answer to all skin problems. In order to make sure that you have nice, healthy and younger looking skin you need to use a variety of products because one skin care product is just not enough.

Almond oil is not only suitable for all skin types but it also provides you with the solution of all the major skin problems. Almond oil contains vitamin E that is excellent to curb early signs of aging and protect skins from, sunburns.

So now there is no need to spend big bucks on anti-aging and sunscreens because you can achieve much better results just by using almond oil.

## Benefits

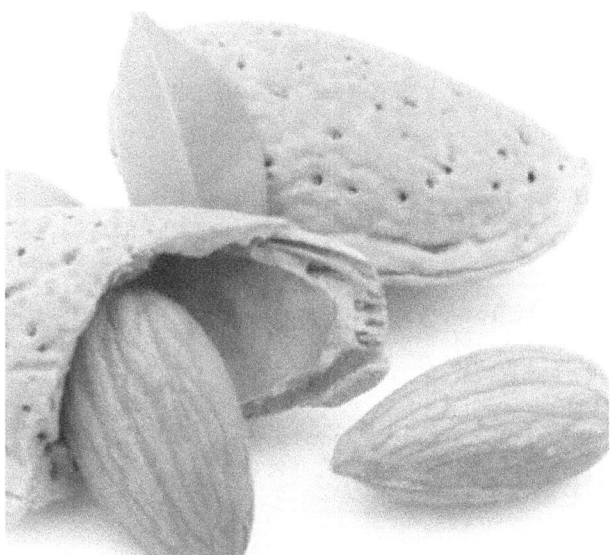

Almond oil is a dream come true for all those people who suffer from a variety of skin problems. Here are some of the benefits that you can avail by using almond oil:

1. Almond oil in an emollient, which means that it nourishes your skin and makes it softer and smoother.

2. It deeply moisturizes your skin.

3. Almond oil controls the aging symptoms on your skin.

4. Almond oil makes you look younger and fresher.

5. Almond oil improves your complexion, giving your skin an even tone.

6. If you have dry and itchy skin then almond oil is the best cure for that.

7. Almond oil is excellent for the treatment of body rashes and chapped lips.

8. Almond oil can be applied to burns to reduce irritation and soreness in the affected area.

9. Almond oil lightens the dark circles around your eyes.

10. Almond oil works as a powerful antioxidant that will keep your skin hydrated.

11. Regular use of almond oil will make your skin look young and fresh.

12. Almond oil contains vitamin E which protects the skin from harmful UV rays.

13. Almond oil helps in reducing the appearance of whiteheads and blackheads on skin.

14. Almond oil can also be used to cure pimples.

15. Almond oil can also be used for taking off make-up, without being harsh on the skin.

## Usage Methods

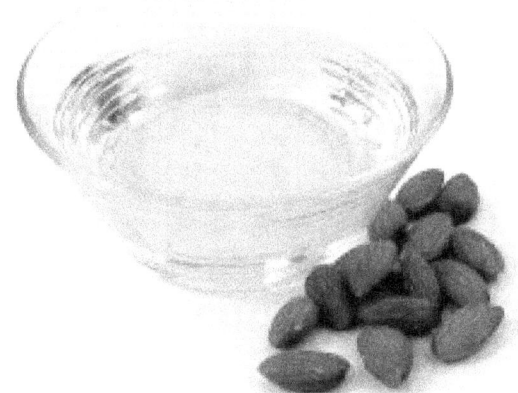

There are several ways of using almond oil on your skin. You can either use it directly or you can also use products that include almond oil as their essential ingredients. Regular use of almonds oil can greatly enhance the health of your skin. Following are some of the ways in which you can apply almond oil on your skin.

## Applying For Wrinkles

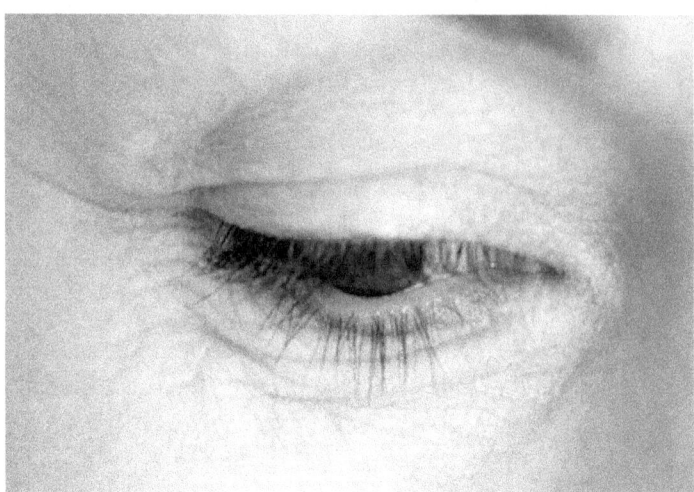

Using almond oil regularly helps in tightening your skin. Applying a coat of almond oil every night will reduce lines and wrinkles on your face.

The best way to apply almond oil is to cleanse your skin before applying a coat of almond oil. Just take a few drops of almond oil on your palm, rub it together and massage it over your face.

## Applying For Dark Circles

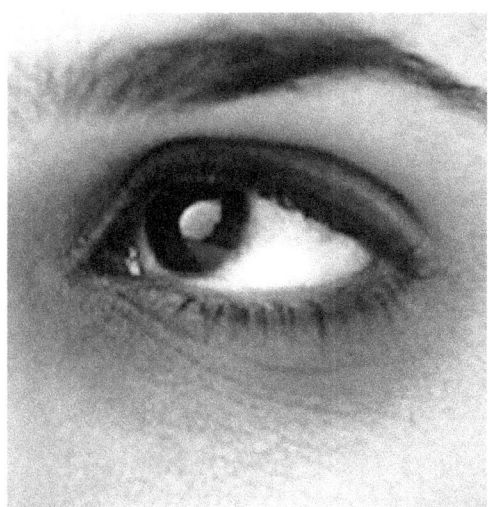

Dark circles make you look dull and tired. Almond oil is very effective in reducing dark circles, making your skin look fresh and young.

For best results add few drops of raw honey in few drops of almond oil and apply on the dark area around the eyes. This mixture will also help in reducing the puffiness around the eyes. Make sure that you apply this very gently as the skin around the eyes is very sensitive and can stretch easily.

## Applying For Eczema and Psoriasis

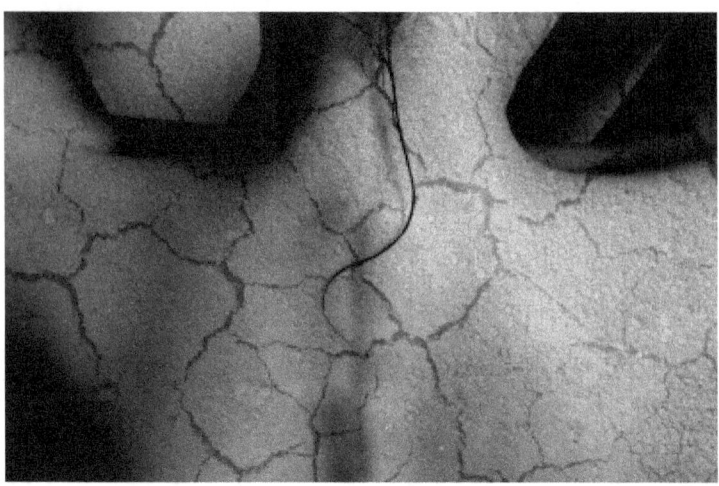

Almond oil has the ability to relieve, skin irritation, inflammation, and itching. Therefore it can be used as a base for eczema and psoriasis treatment.

Add the following to make a mixture:

1. Almond oil 2 tbsp

2. Vitamin E oil 2 drops

3. Chamomile essential oil 5 drops

4. Lavender essential oil 5 drops

Apply this mixture multiple times a day to heal the cracked skin that is caused by eczema and psoriasis.

## Applying For Smooth Skin

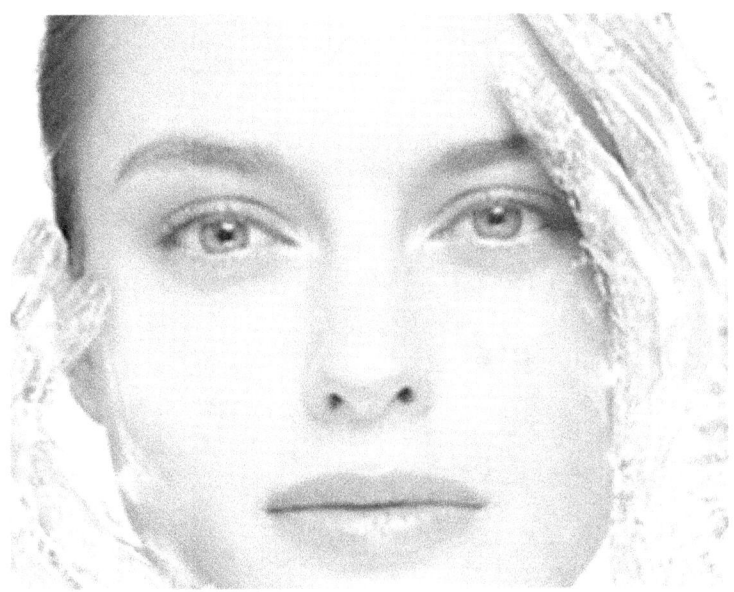

You can use almond oil as a base for sugar scrub for your body and face. To make sugar scrub, mix 1 to 2 tbsp of almond oil with ½ cup of fine sugar.

Apply to your skin and rub gently until your skin starts feeling smoother. Make sure that you avoid the sensitive areas around eyes, and rub your face very carefully to prevent the skin from stretching.

Almond oil is a fantastic cure for many skin problems. It revitalizes and rejuvenates your skin, making you look younger and fresher. Make sure that you are using sweet almond oil, as bitter almond oil is not fit for external or internal use.

Note: Do not use almonds or almond oil if you are allergic to nuts as that might cause severe allergic reaction.

# Nails And Hands

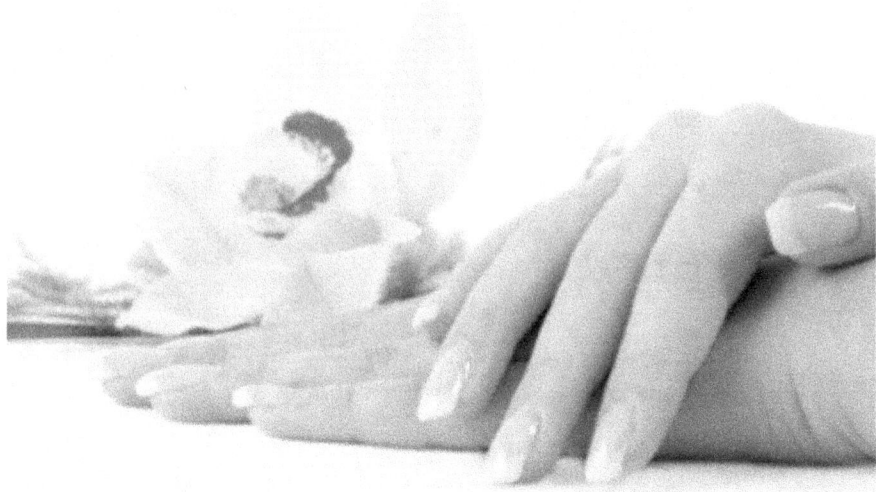

We pay a lot of attention in grooming our face and hair, but we most often neglect our hands and nails. Our hands get exposed to manual work that we do in our day to day activities and yet we do not spend any time in taking care of our hands nails.

Women generally believe that it is only their face and hair that makes them feminine, but in reality hands and nails also add on to the femininity and grace of a woman.

Almond oil is not only good for your face and hair but it is also very effective for your hands and nails. Almond oil is rich in nutrients that help in healing dry and damaged hands and brittle finger nails.

## Benefits

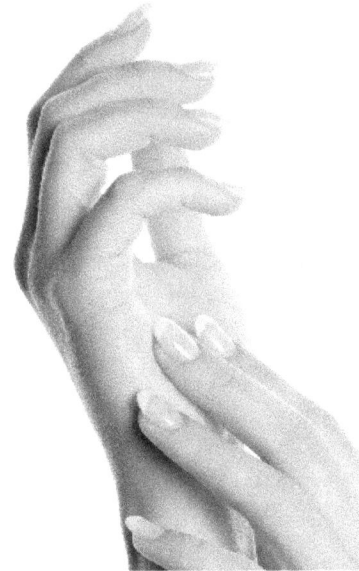

1. Almond oil saves hands from sun damage.

2. With regular use of almond oil the wrinkle and lines on hands are greatly reduced.

3. Almond oil is easily absorbed in your skin; therefore it keeps hand well hydrated without making them oily and slippery.

4. It nourishes, sooths, and moisturizes the dry skin of hands.

5. Almond oil helps in opening clogged pores.

6. It contains zinc which heals wounds and scars faster, without leaving blemishes on skin.

7. Zinc also helps in enhancing the tone and complexion of skin.

8. If your hands are prone to reactions to cleaning products, or you have skin conditions like eczema or psoriasis then almond oil can prove to be of great help because it heals skin faster and soothe irritation and inflammation of skin.

9. Almond oil keeps fingernails nourished and hydrated.

10. Soaking nails in almond oil will keep your nails strong and shiny.

11. Almond oil facilitates faster growth of nails.

12. Almond oil prevents brittle nails, preventing breakage.

## Usage Methods

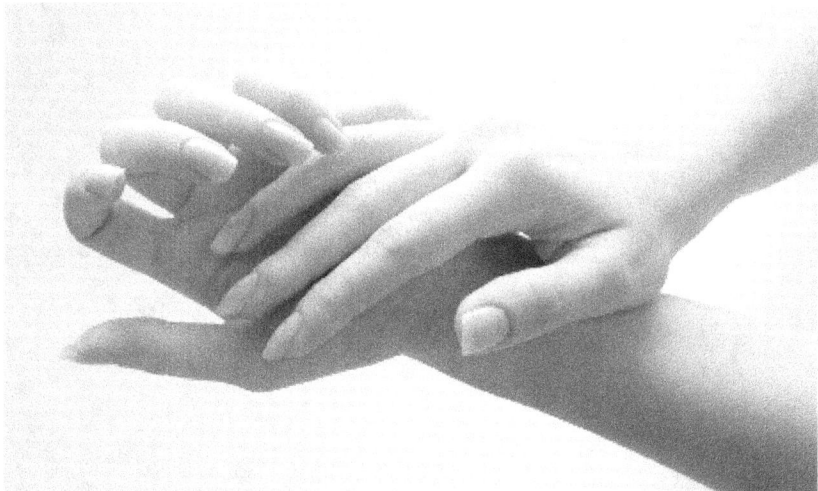

Applying lotions and oil on your skin keeps your hand moisturized and hydrated. However, these products wash off your hand when you are involved in some household chore. Therefore your hands need a product that gets absorbed inside the skin layers and keeps it hydrated even while you are working. Almond oil gets absorbed in your skin and keeps it nourished. Following are some ways in which you can apply almond oil on your hands and nails

## Applying For Smooth Hands

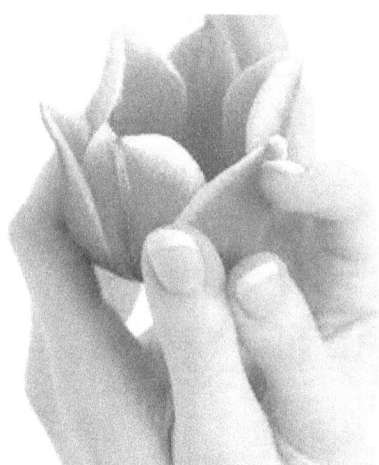

Applying almond oil on hands is fairly simple. Just wash your hand and pour 3 to 4 drops of almond oil on your hands and massage well until it is absorbed in your skin.

You can also apply almond oil over night so keep your hands hydrated and moisturized.

## Applying For Soft Hands

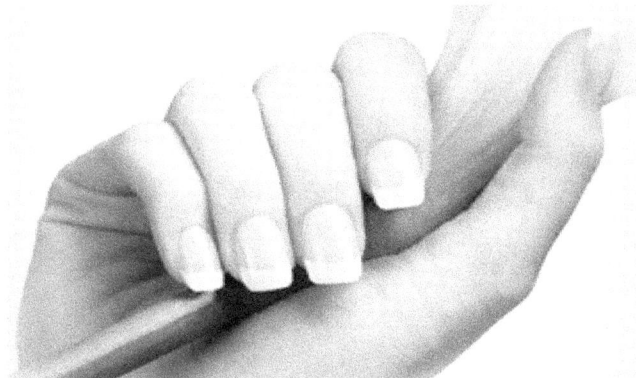

Keeping your hands soft is typically hard. This is because of the work that our hands perform each day. Use sugar scrub on your hands to make your hands soft and to remove dry and dead skin.

Mix ½ cup of fine sugar and add 2 to 3 tbsp of almond oil in it. Rub on your hands gently until you feel your hands becoming smooth and soft.

## Apply For Nails

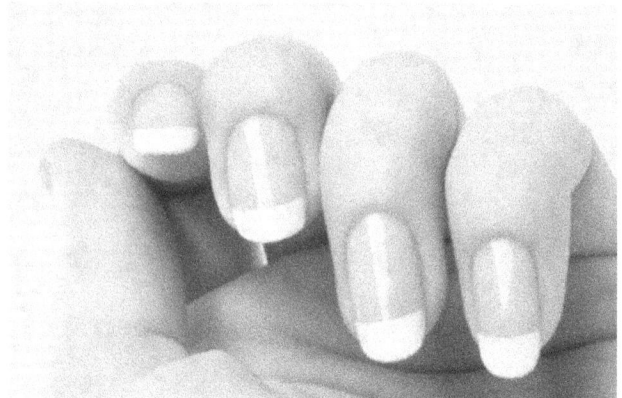

More often than not our nails become too brittle and break easily, which makes it hard for us to keep long, shiny, and strong nails. However, now there is a cure for brittle nails. Almond oil contains minerals that help the nails grow faster without breaking or chipping.

There are two ways of applying almond oil on your nails. You can soak your nails in almond oil once or twice a day to provide them with their required nourishment. You can also use cotton to apply almond oil on your skin. Just dab the cotton in oil and apply it on your nails to get shinier and healthier nails.

# Other Uses And Benefits Of Almond Oil

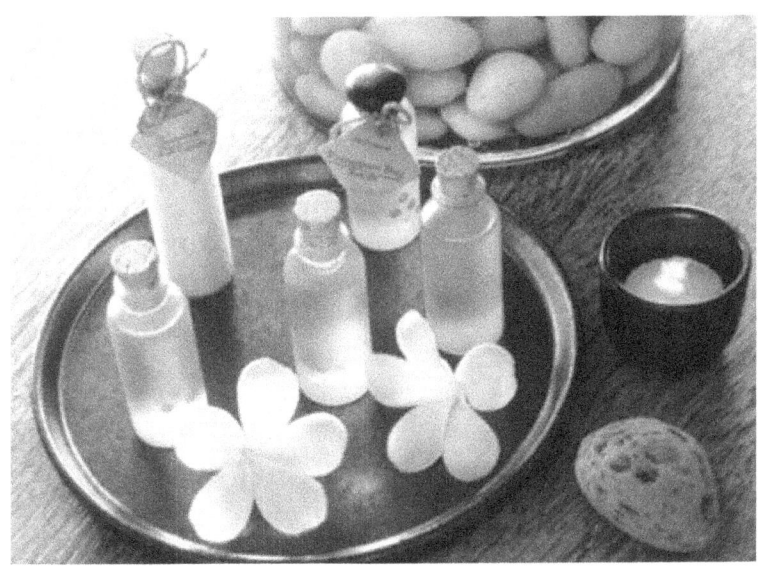

Almond oil is not only beneficial for your hair, skin, hands and nails, but it has many other uses and benefits also. Apart from being a one stop beauty product that is a solution to almost all your beauty problems, almond oil can also be used for following purposes.

## Aromatherapy

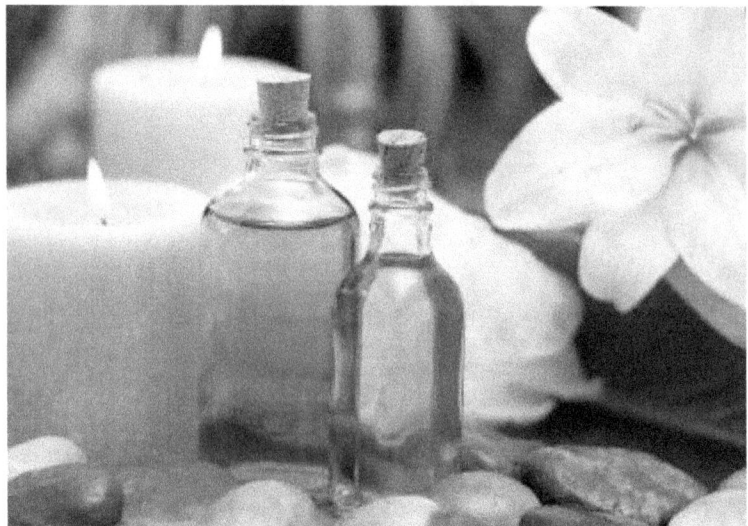

Aromatherapies are used all around the world as alternative medicine that uses a mixture of essential and carrier oils for the purpose of enhancing people's cognitive function, health, moods, and mind.

Almond oil is also used as carrier oil in aromatherapy. Essentials oils are mixed with carrier oils to produce different fragrances and effects. Essential oils are mixed with carriers oils because they can cause irritation on skin if used alone. Almond oil is used as carrier oil because of it is skin friendly and has a sweet smell of almonds.

## Massage Therapy

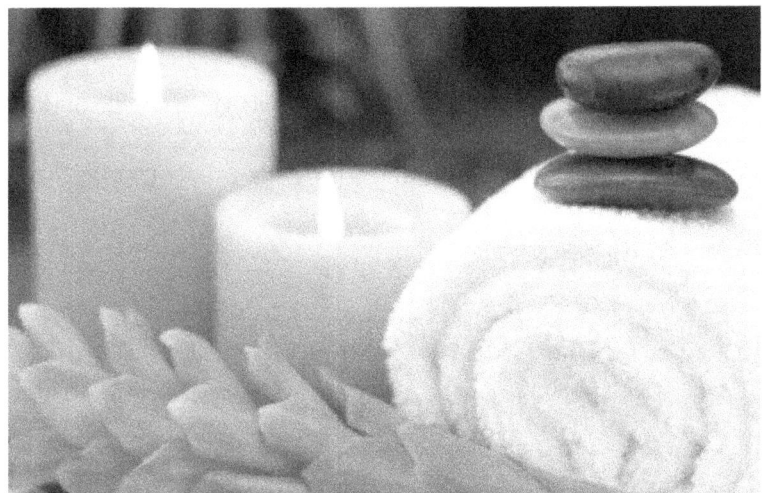

Massage therapy is the manipulation of soft tissues of the body and it consists of fixed pressures and movements that help relieve stress and pain in body muscles.

Almond oil is commonly used for massages around the world because it gets easily absorbed in skin and is suitable for all skin types. Almond oil does not only maintain the moisture of the skin but it also contains fatty acids, linoleic and oleic, that helps in reducing the muscle pains and relieves stress in body and muscles.

# Miracles of Almond

Almond is nothing less than a miracle nut and has been used by various cultures for centuries. It is believed to have multiple benefits and it is considered a drop of life. Following are some of the benefits of almond oil that has been witnessed and experienced by many people over the centuries:

1. 4 to 5 almonds every day is believed to improve the capabilities of brain in children and adults.

2. Almond oil is considered as an excellent nutrient for nervous system.

3. It is believed that they increase the intellectual levels and longevity of nervous system.

4. Almonds contain L-carnitine and riboflavin that boost brain activity.

5. Their memory improving quality decreases the risk of Alzheimer's disease.

6. It has phenylalanine which has the capacity of improving cognitive functions and moods.

7. These nutrients are quick to get absorbed by the brain and help in the production of hormones such as dopamine and adrenaline.

8. These hormones improve brain function and relax our bodies.

9. Almonds lower the risk of cardiovascular diseases.

10. They are rich in Vitamin E that improves the flow of blood.

11. It helps in carrying essential nutrients to different organs in the body.

12. Use of almond oil reduces the risk of blockage in arteries.

13. Almond oil is rich in magnesium that plays a very important role in converting sugar into energy.

14. By adding almonds and almond oil in your diet will help you lose pounds.

15. Eating almonds reduces the risk of gallstones.

16. Almonds improve digestive health.

17. They have pre-biotic qualities that are known to increase the level of useful gut bacteria.

18. Eating almonds also helps in reducing the pain which is beneficial for people with Parkinson's.

19. Since almonds are loaded with folic acid, they are very good for pregnant women.

20. Folic acid helps in the growth of the fetus.

21. Eating 4 to 5 almonds a day helps with constipation.

22. Almonds are like instant capsule of energy because they get quickly absorbed in blood.

23. They are rich in phosphorus and calcium that help in making bones grow stronger in both children and adults.

# Health Benefits of Almond Oil

After mentioning the list of beauty benefits that you can derive from almond oil, it is time to mention the health benefits that you will get by adding almond oil in your diet. Following are some of the innumerable benefits of using almond oil in your recipes:

1. Using oil extracted from nuts reduces the risk of developing cardiovascular diseases.

2. Using almond oil improves the level of cholesterol in your blood.

3. Use of almond oil also improves the health of your colon.

4. Adding almond oil in your diet decreases the chances of colon cancer.

5. Adding almond oil in your diet will help you make up for vitamin E deficiency in your body.

6. Vitamin E protects the cells inside the body from damage and provides protection against chronic diseases such as cancer and cardiac diseases.

7. Vitamin E also improves the immune system.

8. Edible almond oil is high in monounsaturated fats.

9. Can be cooked at high temperatures up to 495°F.

10. Almond oil is a brilliant source of minerals, calcium and healthy fats.

11. Almond oil is rich in Vitamin 1, B6, B2, and B1.

12. Frying and sautéing vegetable in almond oil will add a delicious nutty flavor to your dish without adding more calories.

# Recipes using Almond Oil

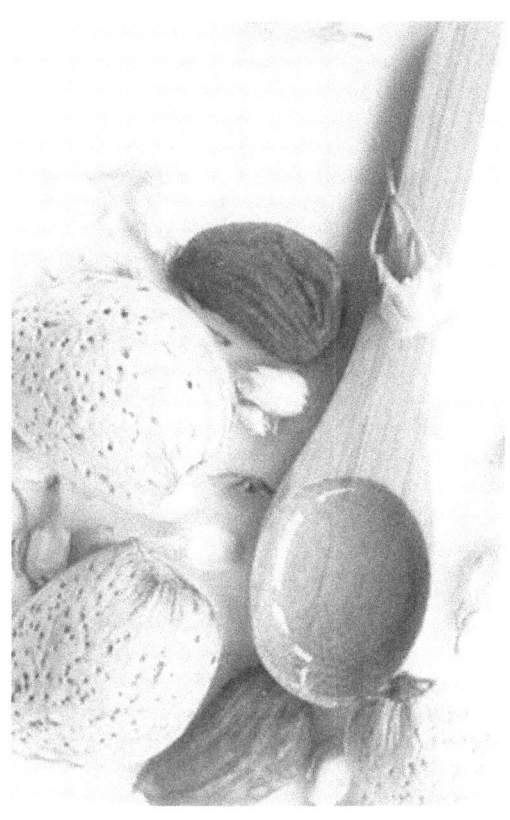

Edible almond oil is very beneficial for health. Cooking dishes in almond oil will not only add nutritional value in your meals but you will also witness the health of your skin, hair, hands, and nails improving over time.

Here are some recipes that you can try toad almond oil in your diet. It will make your dishes more delicious by giving them a nutty flavor and is best for salads and baking cookies and cakes.

## Blood Orange and Arugula Salad

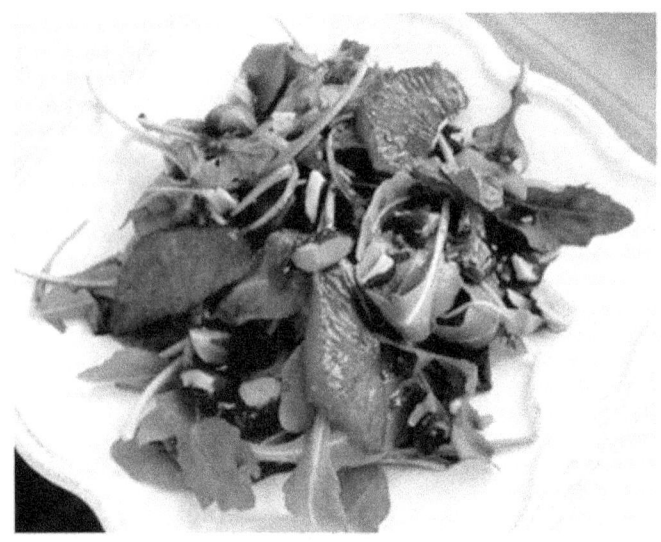

**Serving:** 4

**Nutritional Information (per serving):** K calories 350, carbohydrates 61(g), proteins 4(g), saturates 1(g), fats 14(g), fiber 7(g)

**Ingredients**

1. Arugula 6 cups

2. Blood oranges 2

3. Almonds ½ cup

4. Dates 12

5. Cheese

6. Almond oil (pure) 3 tbsp

7. Salt to taste

8. Black pepper (freshly ground) to taste

## Directions

1. Slice the blossom ends and stems from blood orange.

2. Peel the fruit with you knife and remove the white pith.

3. When you have peeled the oranges, slice the oranges in 7 to 10 pinwheels.

4. Remove the pits of dates and cut in half lengthwise.

5. Place the cheese on a cutting board and shave 16 thin and large slices of cheese with the help of a peeler or  chef's knife

6. Take a large platter and splatter 1/3 or arugula on it.

7. Arrange 1/3 of dates, oranges, nuts and cheese over arugula.

8. Scatter the next layer of arugula and continue scattering layers one over another.

9. This will allow the ingredients to mix well.

10. Sprinkle almond oil on top of these ingredients.

11. Season with pepper, salt, and juice of blood orange.

## Chicken Nuggets

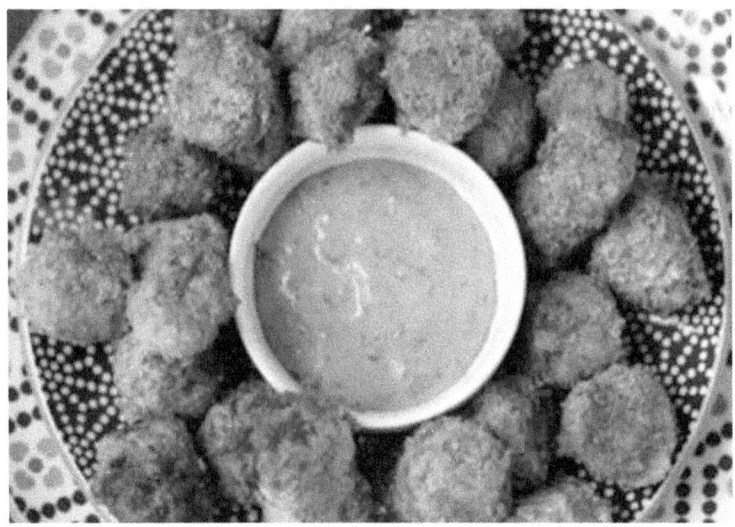

**Serving:** 2

**Nutritional Information (per serving):** K calories 120, carbohydrates 6(g), proteins 2(g), saturates 1.5(g), fats 11(g), fiber 4(g)

**Ingredients**

1. Chicken breast (boneless and skinless) 2

2. Almond oil 1-3 tablespoon

3. Almond meal ½ cup

4. Paprika 1 teaspoon

5. Seasoning (poultry) 1 teaspoon

6. Salt to taste

7. Pepper (ground and fresh) to taste

**Directions**

1. Preheat the oven to 400°F.

2. Generously coat a baking sheet with almond oil and place the pan in oven to heat.

3. Trim the fat from chicken breast then slice each chicken breast in to 5 pieces of nuggets.

4. Pound the pieces to get same thickness.

5. Mix almond meal, poultry seasoning, paprika, pepper, and salt in a bowl and combine will.

6. Coat each nugget with the mixture of almond meal.

7. Marinate all the nuggets before you taking out the baking sheet that was being heated in the oven.

8. Lay all the coated nuggets on the sheet and place them in the oven for around 8 to 10 minutes.

9. Remove from the oven when the nuggets start turning light brown from one side and turn the nuggets to cook from the other side.

10. Serve hot with the sauce of your choice.

# Almond Streusel and Blueberry Muffins

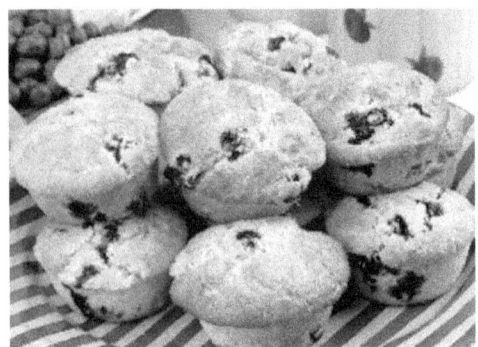

**Serving:** 15

**Nutritional Information (per serving):** K calories 240, carbohydrates 43(g), proteins 6(g), saturates 1.5(g), fats 5(g), fiber 2(g)

## Ingredients for Muffins

1. Flour (divided) 1½ cups
2. Wheat flour 1 cup
3. Oats 1 cup
4. Sugar 1 cup
5. Baking soda 1 teaspoon
6. Salt ¼ teaspoon
7. Vanilla yogurt (low fat) 2 cups
8. Almond oil 3 tablespoons
9. Vanilla extract 2 teaspoons
10. Egg (normal) 1
11. Fresh blueberries 1½ cups
12. Cooking spray

**Ingredients for Streusel**

1. Flour ¼ cup

2. Chopped almonds ¼ cups

3. Brown sugar 1 tablespoon

4. Butter (melted) 1 tablespoon

**Directions for Muffins**

1. Heat the oven to 400 degrees.

2. Measure cups in measuring cups and use a knife to level.

3. Combine flour, oats, wheat flour, sugar, baking soda, baking powder, and salt in a large mixing bowl.

4. Use a whisk to stir.

5. Combine milk, yogurt, oil, egg, and vanilla and stir with a whisk.

6. Add milk and yogurt mixture with flour and mic until moist.

7. Add blueberries.

8. Coat the muffin cups with cooking spray.

9. Add two spoons of batter into muffin cups.

**Direction for Streusel**

1. Combine flour with brown sugar, almonds, and melted butter.

2. Add this mixture on top of each muffin.

3. Place in preheated oven.

4. Bake for around 15 minutes or when muffins start bouncing back when pressed in middle.

5. Take out of oven and let them cool for 10 minutes.

6. Serve at room temperature or warm.

# Chicken and Red Cabbage Salad with Dressing of Cilantro

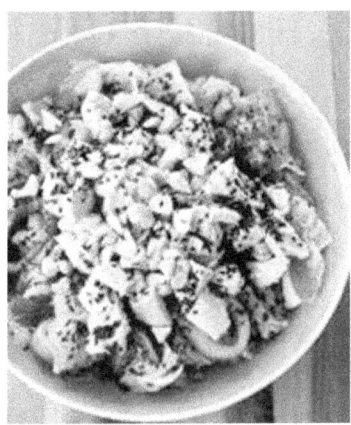

**Serving:** 4

**Nutritional Information (per serving):** K calories 450, carbohydrates 52(g), proteins 19(g), saturates 4(g), fats 22(g), fiber 7(g)

**Ingredients for Dressing**

1. Minced ginger (fresh) ½ teaspoon

2. Minced garlic (fresh) ½ teaspoon

3. Chopped cilantro (fresh) ¼ cup

4. Peanut butter 3 tablespoons

5. Lemon juice 1 tablespoon

6. Peanut oil 2 tablespoons

7. Soy sauce 3 tablespoons

8. Hot water 1 tablespoon

9. Sugar 1 tablespoon

**Ingredients for Salad**

1. Sliced red cabbage 2-3 cups

2. Combination of vegetables of your choice ½ - 1 cup

3. Sliced green onions  (diagonally) 1/3 cup

4. Cooked chicken (diced) 1-2 cups

**Ingredients for Garnish**

1. Chopped cilantro (fresh) 2-3

2. Chopped almonds ¼ cup

3. Almond oil 1 tablespoon

**Directions**

1.  Add garlic, ginger, sugar, hot water, soy sauce, lemon juice, almond oil, peanut butter, cilantro in a processor.

2.  Process for around a minute until all the ingredients mix well.

3.  Take out the outer leaves of the cabbage.

4.  Cut the core out and chop into thin slices.

5.  Chop other vegetables into thick slices.

6.  Cut chicken into squares of 1 inch.

7.  Take a salad bowl and add all the vegetables and chicken in it.

8.  Mix with dressing.

9.  Take out in separate plates and decorate with almond oil, chopped cilantro and almonds.

# Crispy Almond Flour Cheese Crackers

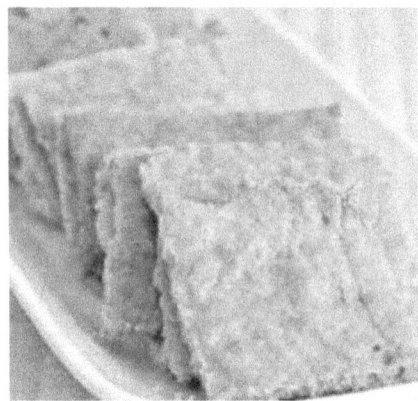

**Serving:** 4

**Nutritional Information (per serving):** K calories 240, carbohydrates 30(g), proteins 7(g), saturates 3.5(g), fats 10(g), fiber 1(g)

**Ingredients**

1. Almond flour 1¼ cups

2. Salt 1/8 teaspoon

3. Baking soda ¼ teaspoon

4. Cheddar cheese (grated) ½ cup

5. Almond oil 1½ tablespoon

6. Egg (large) 1

**Directions**

1. Heat the oven at 350°f.

2. Add almond flour, baking soda, salt, and cheese in a medium sized mixing bowl.

3. Take another bowl and whish egg and oil together.

4. Add the mixture of egg and oil with almond flour and mix well.

5. Take parchment paper and cut it in the size of your baking sheet.

6. Put the parchment paper on an even surface and place the dough over it.

7. Put the second piece of parchment of top of the dough and use a rolling pin to roll the dough.

8. Make sure that you roll the dough in such a way that it is of even thickness on all sides.

9. Remove the top parchment and cut in squares of 2 inches.

10. Place the parchment on baking sheet and place in oven

11. Bake for around 12-15 minutes.

12. Taking out the baking sheet when crackers are light brown in color and let them cool for 20 to 30 minutes,

13. Keep the crackers in a plastic container to save them from going stale.

## Conclusion

Almond oil has been in use for centuries and it benefits are now medically proven. It is nothing less than magic in a flask. Almond oil is one stop solution for many beauty and health issues that we face in our daily life.

It is time that you stop spending big bucks on expensive beauty products because you will find the answer to all your beauty related issues in almond oil. Not only will it help you become younger, fresher, and more beautiful, but it will also improve your health drastically.

This book not only gives you knowledge about the benefits and uses of almond oil in terms of your beauty, but it also has recipes that are easy to make and are mouth watering treats for your taste buds. Use almond oil on a regular basis and witness a change in your overall health. Become as beautiful on the outside as you are on inside by using this oil with miraculous qualities.